*INSPIRED*
*by the teachings of*

## Swāmī Kuvalayānandaji
## Swāmī Digambarji
## Dr. S.A. Shukla

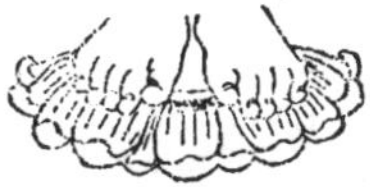

# Acknowledgments

My special thanks to the following for their suggestions, criticism, and/or inspiration

*Dr. M.V. Bhole*
*Shri R.K. Bodhe*
*Lorraine Cahn*
*Dr. G.S. Chhina*
*Philip Davidoff*
*Dr. M.M. Gore*
*Margaret Smith James*
*Dr. P. Jha*
*Barbara Levitt*
*Gershon Levitt*
*Swami Maheshananda*
*Dr. G. Ramakrishna*
*Shri G.S. Sahay*
*Orit Sen-Gupta*
*Dr. B.R. Sharma*
*Candace Smith*
*Swami Shri Sunilananda*
*Shri O.P. Tiwari*

*for my*
*student-teachers*

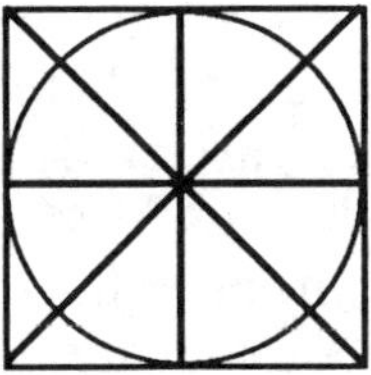

This Mandala includes all their names.

# Introduction

YOGA VISION is the result of my study of the Yoga Sutras at the feet of Swami Kuvalayanandaji and Dr. S.A. Shukla (1959–1961) and later with Swami Digambarji (1966–1990). The co-workers of the Scientific and Philosophical Literary Research Departments of the K.S.M.Y.M. Samiti, Kaivalyadhama, Lonavla also inspired its outcome.

The many years of teaching Yoga and Mental Health to students of the G.S. College of Yoga and Cultural Synthesis, the Summer Camp Certificate Course at Kaivalyadhama, and the students and teachers of SKY Foundation, gave me the insight

3-

# Yoga Vision

## A Selection of Yoga Sutras

Sanskrit Text in Devanagari
with Roman Transliteration
and English Translation

Vijayendra Pratap, Ph.D., D.Y.P.

SKY Foundation
Philadelphia, Pennsylvania, USA

*First Draft, January 14, 1992*
*First printing, May 2, 1995*

*Library of Congress Catalog*
*Card Number 95-068061*
*ISBN 0-944731-01-5*

*Published by*
*Swami Kuvalayananda Yoga (SKY) Foundation*
*339 Fitzwater Street*
*Philadelphia, Pennsylvania 19147 USA*

*Distributed by*
*Garland of Letters Bookstore*
*527 South Street*
*Philadelphia, Pennsylvania, 19147 USA*

*Distributed Overseas by*
*Akash Prakashan*
*12/203 Commercial Complex*
*Preet Vihar, Vikas Marg,*
*New Delhi-110092, INDIA*

*Printed by Science Press*
*Ephrata, Pennsylvania*

to look at the Sutras in a completely different way. This translation reflects that view.

According to the majority of translators, Bhagavan Shri Patanjali compiled 195 Yoga Sutras. Sutra means a thread, string, line, or cord; a collection of threads; an aphorism or short, concise statement. The six qualities of a sutra are defined as:

स्वल्पाक्षरमसंदिग्धं सारवद्विश्वतोमुखम् ।
अस्तोभमनवद्यं च सूत्रं सूत्रविदो विदुः ॥

(1) very few words, (2) clear, fully expressive, (3) having essence, (4) facing all sides, i.e.

having a universal application touching all points, (5) self-sufficient, (6) praiseworthy or fit to be spoken.

Scholars differ widely in estimating Maharishi Patanjali's era. According to Woods, he lived between 300 and 500 AD. Rukmani suggests 200 BC to 100 AD. And Bailey places him between 820 BC and 300 BC, allowing that he may date back as early as 10,000 BC.

While all of the Sutras are very rich in Yogic philosophy and its practice, the 27 Sutras selected for this work cover the essence of Kriya and Astanga Yoga and their practices.

The Yoga Sutras provide a wealth of knowledge which is ever increasing. I dare not claim that I fully understand their message, but I definitely enjoy them. To know their secrets... read, recite, and review them again and again.

And remember, maps are more useful if you travel.

Best Wishes,

Vijay

# TRANSLITERATION

| SAṀSKṚTA | LETTERS | PRONUNCIATION |
|---|---|---|
| अ | a | sun |
| आ | â | art |
| इ | i | sit |
| ई | î | seat |
| उ | u | pull |
| ऊ | û | wool |
| ऋ | ṛ | merrily |
| ए | e | sage |
| ऐ | ai | aisle |
| ओ | o | home |
| औ | au | house |
| ं | ṁ (am) | momentum |
| : | ḥ | hut |

## (IN DEVANÂGARÎ ORDER)

| SAṀSKṚTA | LETTERS | PRONUNCIATION |
|---|---|---|
| क् | k | calm |
| ख् | kh | Eckhart |
| ग् | g | God |
| घ् | gh | ghost |
| ङ् | ṅ | king |
| च् | c | chariot |
| छ् | ch | charge |
| ज् | j | joy |
| झ् | jh | hedgehog |
| ञ् | ñ | Señor |
| ट् | ṭ | twist |
| ठ् | ṭh | anthill |
| ड् | ḍ | devotion |

## TRANSLITERATION

| SAṀSKṚTA | LETTERS | PRONUNCIATION |
|---|---|---|
| ढ् | ḍh | adhere |
| ण् | ṇ | tender |
| त् | t | thin |
| थ् | th | thought |
| द् | d | then |
| ध् | dh | this |
| न् | n | nose |
| प् | p | patience |
| फ् | ph | philosophy |
| ब् | b | bow |
| भ् | bh | abhor |
| म् | m | monk |

## (IN DEVANÂGARÎ ORDER)

| SAṀSKṚTA | LETTERS | PRONUNCIATION |
|---|---|---|
| य् | y | yoke |
| र् | r | road |
| ल् | l | love |
| व् | v | value |
| श् | š | sure |
| ष् | ṣ | shut |
| स् | s | seer |
| ह् | h | hut |
| ळ | ḷ | |
| क्ष् | kṣ | Lakṣmî |
| ज्ञ् | jñ | jñâna |

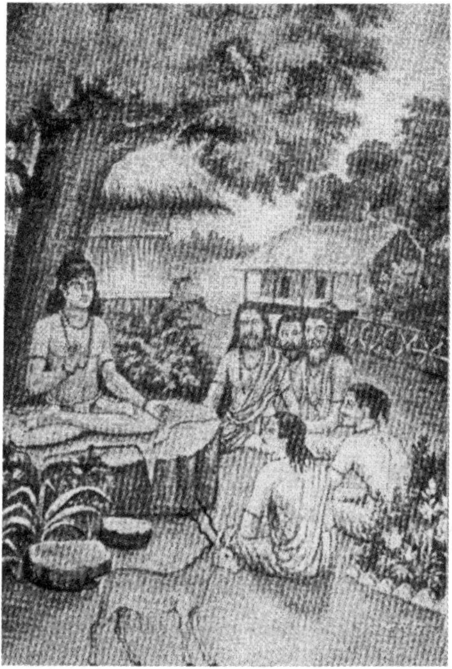

*courtesy of Gita Press*

ॐ

योगेन चित्तस्य पदेन वाचां
मलं शरीरस्य च वैद्यकेन ।
योऽपाकरोत्तं प्रवरं मुनीनां
पतञ्जलिं प्राञ्जलिरानतोऽस्मि ॥

Yogena cittasya, padena vācāṁ
malaṁ śarīrasya ca vāidyakena /
yo 'pākarottaṁ pravaraṁ munīnāṁ
Patañjaliṁ prāñjalirānato 'smi //

I bow with folded hands to
Maharṣi Patañjali, the foremost
thinker who prevented (removed)
the dis-order of consciousness by Yoga,
imperfection of speech by grammar,
and impurity of the body by medicine.

# 1

अथ योगानुशासनम् । (१.१)

atha yogānuśāsanam / I:1

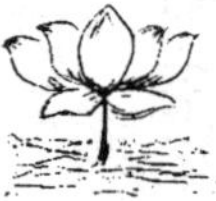

Now a Yoga re-vision (re-teaching).

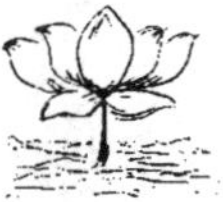

## 2

योगश्चित्तवृत्तिनिरोधः ।

(१.२)

Yogaścitta-vṛtti-nirodhaḥ /
I:2

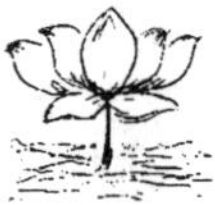

**Yoga is the prevention (control) of dis-order (dis-ease, modifications) of consciousness.**

3

तदा द्रष्टुः
स्वरूपेऽवस्थानम् । (१.३)

tadā draṣṭuḥ
svarūpe avasthānam / I:3

**Then the Observer (Seer) remains in His own form.**

# 4

वृत्तिसारूप्यमितरत्र । (१.४)

vṛtti-sārūpyamitaratra / I:4

Otherwise He is
identified with the
dis-orders (modifications).

## 5

वृत्तयः पञ्चतय्यः
क्लिष्टाक्लिष्टाः । (१.५)

vṛttayaḥ pañcatayyaḥ
kliṣṭākliṣṭāḥ / I:5

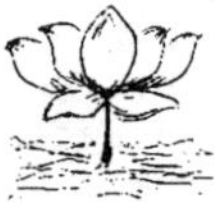

**The mental modifications are fivefold, stressful or non-stressful.**

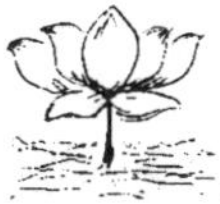

## 6

अभ्यासवैराग्याभ्यां
तन्निरोधः । (१.१२)

abhyāsa-vairāgyābhyāṁ
tannirodhaḥ / I:12

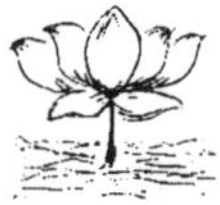

Their prevention (control) is by practice and non-attachment (disinterestedness).

## 7

स तु दीर्घकालनैरन्तर्य
सत्कारासेवितो
दृढभूमिः । (१.१४)

sa tu dīrghakālanairantarya
satkārāsevito
dṛḍhabhūmiḥ/ I:14

**That (practice) becomes established if done for a long time, continuously and with respect.**

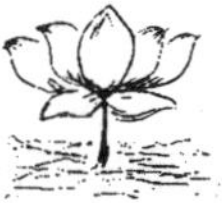

8

ईश्वरप्रणिधानाद्वा ।

(१.२३)

īśvara-praṇidhānādvā /

I:23

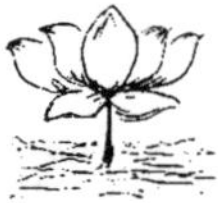

**Or devotion to God.**

9

तस्य वाचकः प्रणवः ।

(१.२७)

tasya vācakaḥ praṇavaḥ /
I:27

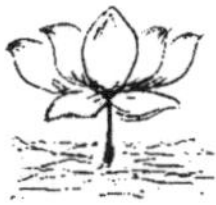

ॐ

**His (God's) name is Praṇava (Om).**

## 10

तज्जपस्तदर्थ
भावनम् । (१.२८)

tajjapastadartha-
bhāvanam / I:28

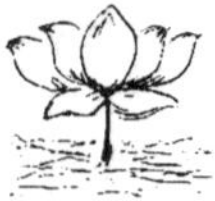

Its (Om) recitation
again and again,
with understanding
and contemplation
on its meaning.

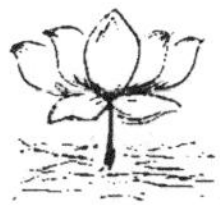

# 11

यथाभिमतध्यानाद्वा ।

(१.३९)

yathābhimata-dhyānādvā /
I:39

**Or meditation on anything (uplifting) of one's choice.**

## 12

तपःस्वाध्यायेश्वर
प्रणिधानानि क्रियायोगः ।

(२.१)

tapaḥ-svādhyāyeśvara-
praṇidhānāni kriyāyogaḥ /
II:1

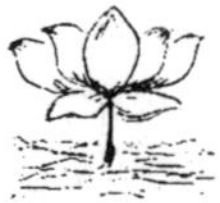

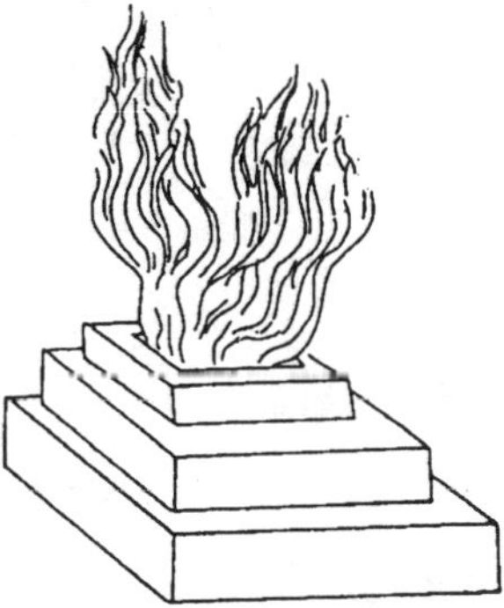

**Simple living (Prāṇāyāma), self-study (recitation), surrender (worship) to God constitute Kriyā Yoga.**

## 13

समाधिभावनार्थः
क्लेशतनूकरणार्थश्च ।

(२.२)

samādhi-bhāvanārthaḥ
kleśa-tanūkaraṇārthaśca /
II:2

**For the integration (of personality) and weakening the stressors (Kleśas).**

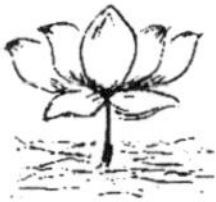

## 14

यमनियमासन

प्राणायामप्रत्याहार

धारणाध्यान

समाधयोऽष्टावङ्गानि ।

(२.२९)

yama-niyama-āsana-
prāṇāyāma-pratyāhāra-
dhāraṇā-dhyāna-
samādhayo'ṣṭāvaṅgāni /

II:29

**Self-regulation,**
**observances,**
**posture,**
**breath regulation,**
**sense withdrawal,**
**concentration,**
**meditation,**
**integration**
**are the eight limbs**
**of Yoga.**

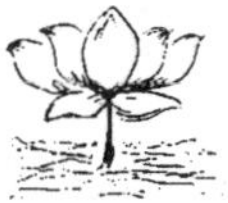

## 15

अहिंसासत्यास्तेय
ब्रह्मचर्यापरिग्रहा
यमाः । (२.३०)

ahiṁsā-satya-asteya-
brahmacarya-aparigrahā -
yamāḥ / II:30

**Non-violence
(Compassion),
truthfulness,
non-stealing,
great conduct,
non-possessiveness
constitute
self-regulations.**

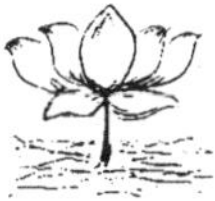

## 16

शौचसन्तोषतपः
स्वाध्यायेश्वर
प्रणिधानानि नियमाः ।

(२.३२)

śauca-santoṣa-tapaḥ-
svādhyāya-īśvara-
praṇidhānāni niyamāḥ /
II:32

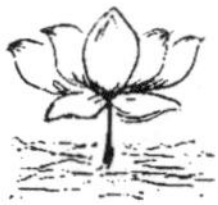

**Cleanliness,**
**contentment,**
**austerity (simple living),**
**self-study (recitation),**
**trust in God**
**constitute observances.**

17

स्थिरसुखमासनम् ।

(२.४६)

sthira-sukham-āsanam /
II:46

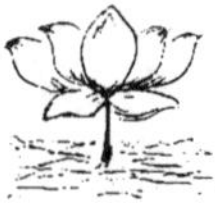

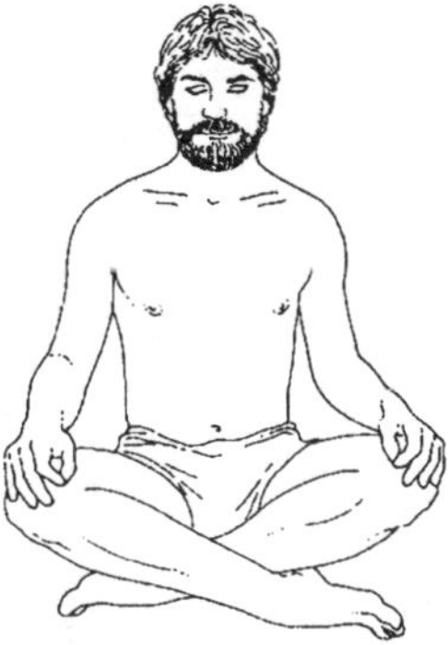

**Stable and comfortable (sense of well-being) is the posture.**

18

ततो द्वन्द्वानभिघातः ।

(२.४८)

tato dvandvānabhighātaḥ /

II:48

**Then no disturbance**
**rom conflicting impulses.**

## 19

तस्मिन्सति
श्वासप्रश्वासयोर्गति
विच्छेदः प्राणायामः ।

(२.४९)

tasmin-sati
śvāsa-praśvāsayor-gati-
vicchedaḥ prāṇāyāmaḥ /
II:49

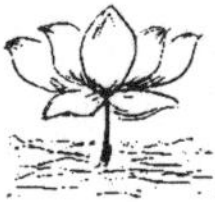

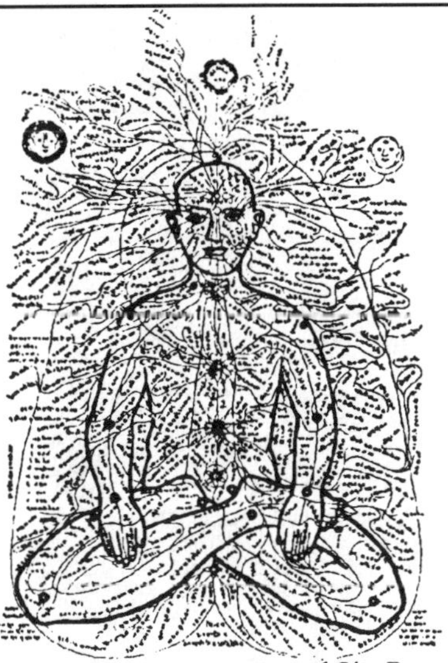

*courtesy of Gita Press*

**After this, regulation (cessation of movement) of inhalation and exhalation is Prāṇāyāma.**

20

ततः क्षीयते
प्रकाशावरणम् । (२.५२)

tataḥ kṣīyate
prakāśāvaraṇam / II:52

**Then disappearance of the covering on the (inner) light.**

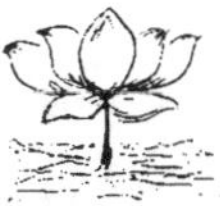

## 21

धारणासु च योग्यता
मनसः । (२.५३)

dhāraṇāsu ca yogyatā
manasaḥ / II:53

**And the mind develops the ability (fitness) to focus.**

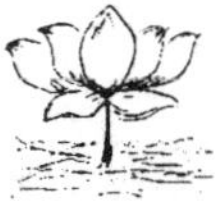

## 22

स्वविषयासंप्रयोगे
चित्तस्वरूपानुकार
इवेन्द्रियाणां
प्रत्याहारः । (२.५४)

sva-viṣayāsaṁprayoge
citta-svarūpānukāra
ivendriyāṇāṁ
pratyāhāraḥ / II:54

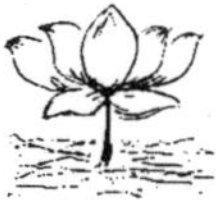

There is no contact with
the objects of perception,
the consciousness is in
its own self (form),
this is the withdrawal
of the senses.

23

देशबन्धश्चित्तस्य
धारणा । (३.१)

deśa-bandhaścittasya
dhāraṇā / III:1

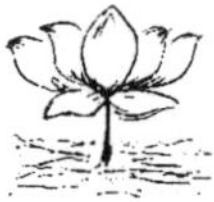

**The fixation of consciousness in (this) space is concentration.**

## 24

तत्र प्रत्ययैकतानता
ध्यानम् । (३.२)

tatra pratyayaikatānatā
dhyānam /III:2

**Then the stretch of consciousness (continuous flow) in the same space is meditation.**

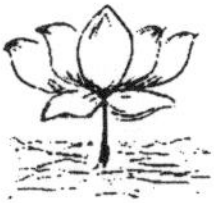

## 25

तदेवार्थमात्रनिर्भासं
स्वरूपशून्यमिव
समाधिः । (३.३)

tadevārthamātra-nirbhāsaṁ
svarūpa-śūnyamiva
samādhiḥ / III:3

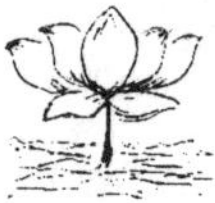

**Then only the**
**consciousness of the same**
**remains,**
**as if oneself were lost,**
**is Samādhi (integration).**

## 26

त्रयमन्तरङ्गं
पूर्वेभ्यः । (३.७)

trayam antaraṅgaṁ
pūrvebhyaḥ / III:7

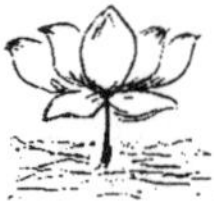

**These three (Dhāraṇā, Dhyāna, Samādhi) constitute the inner (intimate) Yoga in relation to the preceding (Yama, Niyama,Āsana, Prāṇāyāma, Pratyāhāra).**

27

तदपि बहिरङ्गं
निर्बीजस्य । (३.८)

tadapi bahiraṅgaṁ
nirbījasya / III:8

**Even this (Samādhi) is external compared to consciousness without object (Nirbīja Samādhi).**

# A Short Bibliography

Aprabuddha, Shree (1988). The Science of Yoga. Nagpur, India: Shree Aprabuddha Vichar-Sadhana.

Apte, Vaman Shivram (1890). The Student's Sanskrit-English Dictionary. Delhi, India: Shri Jainendra Press.

Āraṇya, Swāmī Hariharānanda (1963). Yoga Philosophy of Patañjali. Calcutta, India: Calcutta University Press.

Baba, Bangali (1976). The Yogasūtra of Patañjali with the Commentary of Vyāsa. Delhi, India: Motilal Banarsidass.

Bailey, Alice A. (1927). The Light of the Soul. Its Science and Effect. A Paraphrase of The Yoga Sutras of Patanjali. New York, NY: Lucis Publishing Company.

Baxi, Vishnuprasad V. (1965). Yoga Darshana. Patanjali. Monghyr. (Bihar), India: Bihar School of Yoga.

Collins, Mabel (1912). The Transparent Jewel. London, Great Britain: William Rider & Son, Ltd.

Coster, Geraldine (1934). Yoga and Western Psychology. A Comparison. London, Great Britain: Oxford University Press.

D'Andrade, Hugh (1971). The Royal Yoga. A Free Translation of the Sutras of Patanjali. New York, NY: Samuel Weiser Inc.

Digambarji, Swami (1987). Transliteration and Easy Rendering of Patanjali's Yoga Sutras. Kaivalyadhama. Lonavla, India: SKY, Number 14.

Digambarji, Swami and Sahai, Dr. Mahajot (1972-1973). Yoga Kośa. Yoga Terms explained with Reference to Context. (Vols. 1-2). Lonavla, India: Kaivalyadhama S. M. Y. M. Samiti.

Dvivedi, M.N. (1890). The Yoga-Sūtras of Patanjali. Delhi, India: Sri Satguru Publications.

Elenjimittam, Anthony (1974). The Yoga Philosophy of Patanjali. Allahabad, India: Allahabad Saint Paul Society.

Eliade, Mircea (1907). Patanjali and Yoga. New York, NY: Schocken Books.

Feuerstein, Georg (1979). The Yoga-Sūtra of Patañjali. Rochester, Vermont: Inner Traditions International, Ltd.

Giri, Swami Satyeswarananda Maharaj (1987). Inner Victory. Vol. 4. San Diego, CA: The Sanskrit Classics.

Jha, Ganganatha (1934). The Yoga-Darshana. The Sutras of Patanjali - with the Bhasya of Vyasa. Adyar, Madras, India: Theosophical Publishing House.

Johnston, Charles (1912). The Yoga Sutras of Patanjali. The Book of the Spiritual Man. London, Great Britain: Watkins Publishing.

Judge, William Q. (1885). The Yoga Aphorisms of Patanjali. Los Angeles, California: The Theosophy Company.

Karambelkar, Dr. P.V. (1987). Pātanjala Yoga Sutras. Sanskrit Sutra with Transliteration, Translation & Commentary. Lonavla, India: Kaivalyadhāma.

Kuvalayānanda, Swāmī (est. 1924). Yoga Mīmāṁsā. A Quarterly Journal devoted to Scientific and Philosophico-Literary Research. Lonavla, India: Kaivalyadhāma.

Leggett, Trevor (1981-1983). Śaṅkara on the Yoga-Sūtras. Vol. I: Samādhi. Vol II: Means. London, Great Britain: Routledge & Kegan Paul, Ltd.

Mehta, Rohit (1975). Yoga: The Art of Integration. A Commentary on the Yoga Sutras of Patanjali. Adyar, Madras, India: The Theosophical Publishing House.

Mishra, Rammurti S., M.D. (1963). Yoga Sutras. The Textbook of Yoga Psychology. Garden City, New York: Anchor Books, Anchor Press/ Doubleday.

Prabhavananda, Swami and Isherwood, Christopher (1953). How to Know God. The Yoga Aphorisms of Patanjali. Hollywood, California: Vedanta Press.

Prasada, Rama (1924). Patanjali's Yoga Sutras. Allahabad, India: Subhindranath Vasu.

Rajneesh, Bhagwan Shree (1976-1978). Yoga: the alpha and the omega. Discourses on the Yoga Sutras of Patanjali (Vols. 1–10). Poona, India: Rajneesh Foundation.

Rukmani, T.S. (1980). Yogavārttika of Vijñānabhikṣu. New Delhi, India: Munshiram Manoharlal Publishers Pvt. Ltd.

Sadhakas (1975). Patanjali's Yoga Sutra. Bombay, India: The Yoga Sadhak Group.

Satchidananda, Sri Swami (1978). Integral Yoga. The Yoga Sutras of Patanjali. Pomfret Center, Connecticut: Integral Yoga Publications.

Swāmi, Shree Purohit (1938). Aphorisms of Yoga by Bhagwān Shree Patanjali. London, Great Britain: Faber & Faber, Ltd.

Taimni, I.K. (1961). The Science of Yoga. The Yoga– Sūtras of Patañjali. Adyar, Madras, India: The Theosophical Publishing House.

Vivekānanda, Swāmi (1897). Rāja-Yoga. Conquering the Internal Nature. Calcutta, India: Advaita Ashrama.

Vivekānanda, Swāmī (1897). Rāja Yoga and Other Subjects. Also Patanjali's Yoga Aphorisms, with Commentaries, and Glossary of Sanskrit Terms. New York, NY: The Baker & Taylor Co.

Woods, James Haughton (1914). The Yoga-System of Patañjali. Or the Ancient Hindu Doctrine of Concentration of Mind. Delhi, India: Motilal Banarsidass *(Authorized Reprint).*

Yardi, M.R. (1979). The Yoga of Patañjali. Poona, India: Bhandarkar Oriental Research Institute.

NOTE

Diacritical marks in the bibliography follow the typesetting of the original texts.